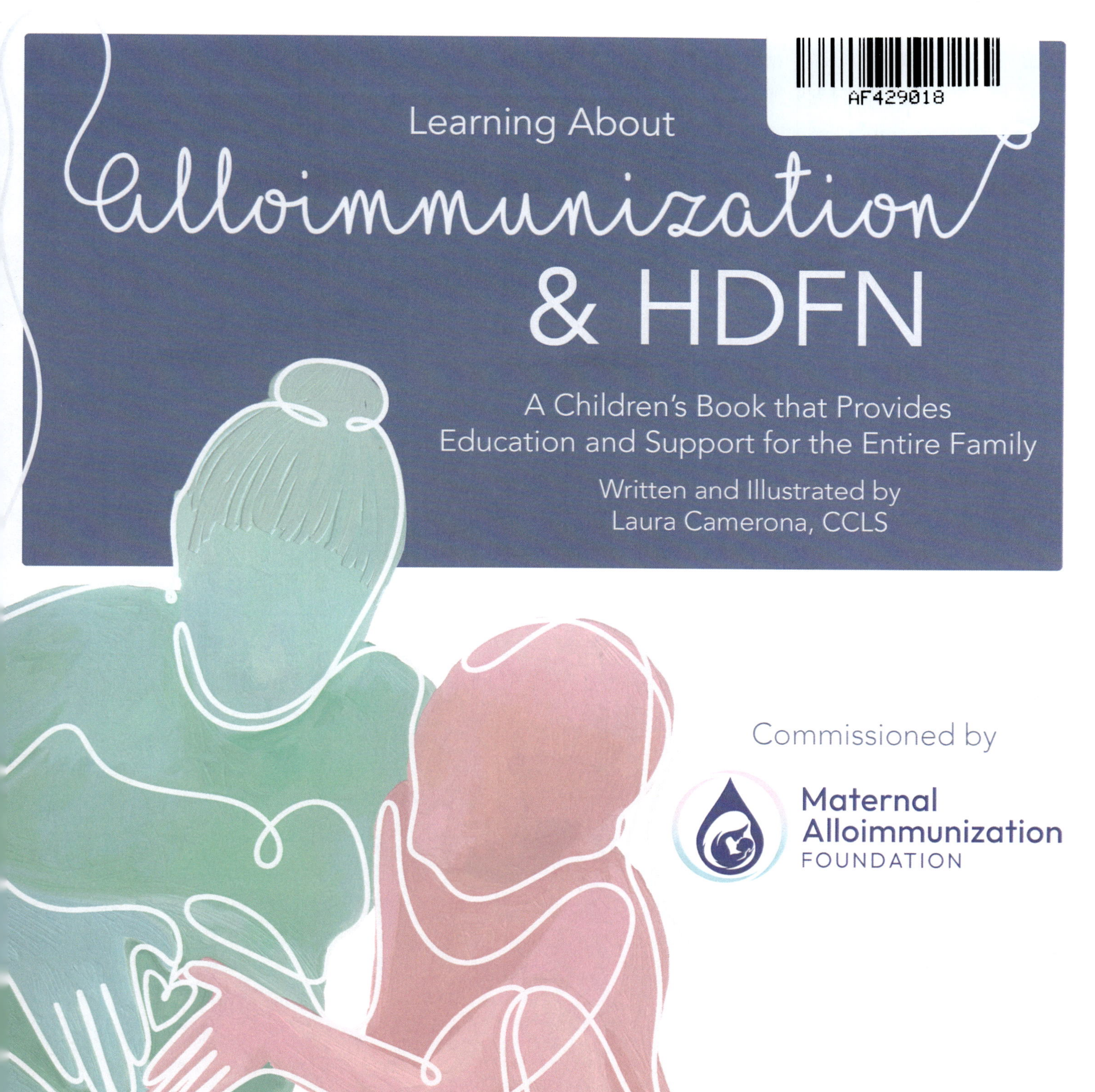

Learning About
Alloimmunization & HDFN
A Children's Book that Provides
Education and Support for the Entire Family
Written and Illustrated by
Laura Camerona, CCLS
Commissioned by
Maternal Alloimmunization FOUNDATION
AF429018

Library of Congress Control Number: 2026936502

This book was written to be appropriate for a wide range of ages.
Each caregiver should use their own knowledge
of their children and the tips provided on the next page to decide
when to read this book with their children. Some families may choose
to only read parts to their children, avoiding the extra detail boxes.

ISBN Paperback: 979-8-9921012-8-7

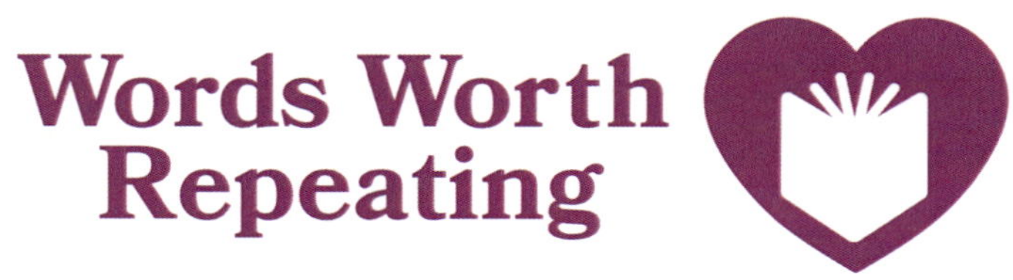

www.wordsworthrepeating.com

Des Moines, IA

Tips for Adults Before Reading This Book:

-This book was written for an adult caregiver to read with a child. This is not a book to just hand to a child if they haven't read it before. Children will often have questions and need support processing all of the information and how it impacts their own family.

-Read this book on your own before reading it with a child. Most children thrive when given honest information in a gentle, non-scary manner, but you are the expert on your child. If some of the information seems like too much for your situation or your child, skip pages or just read the big text and not the small boxes. The book can be reread with more details when your child is ready for them or when you know more about your personal situation.

-Follow your child's lead. If your child wants to take a break after a couple of pages, that is okay. Give them opportunities to come back to it later.

-Emotions are okay. If you get emotional when reading this book, that is okay. Just explain your emotions in simple words. When kids see you being emotional, it shows them that they don't have to cover up their own feelings. Make sure they know that however they feel is okay, even if their emotions don't match yours.

-If your child acts disinterested, this is okay and normal. A lot of the time, kids are listening even if it doesn't seem like it. Let them know if they ever want to come back with questions, that is okay. You might be surprised about the things they will ask once given the time to process.

-This book was written with kids in mind, but also with the idea that even adults can benefit from things being explained in a simple manner. If there are adults in your life that are having a hard time understanding maternal alloimmunization and all of the care involved, this book can be used as a tool for them as well.

-If you are looking for further support in your maternal alloimmunization journey, don't hesitate to reach out to the Maternal Alloimmunization Foundation.
www.alloimmunization.com

In honor of all of our HDFN babies, especially Louise.
Your lives will continue to light the way for others.

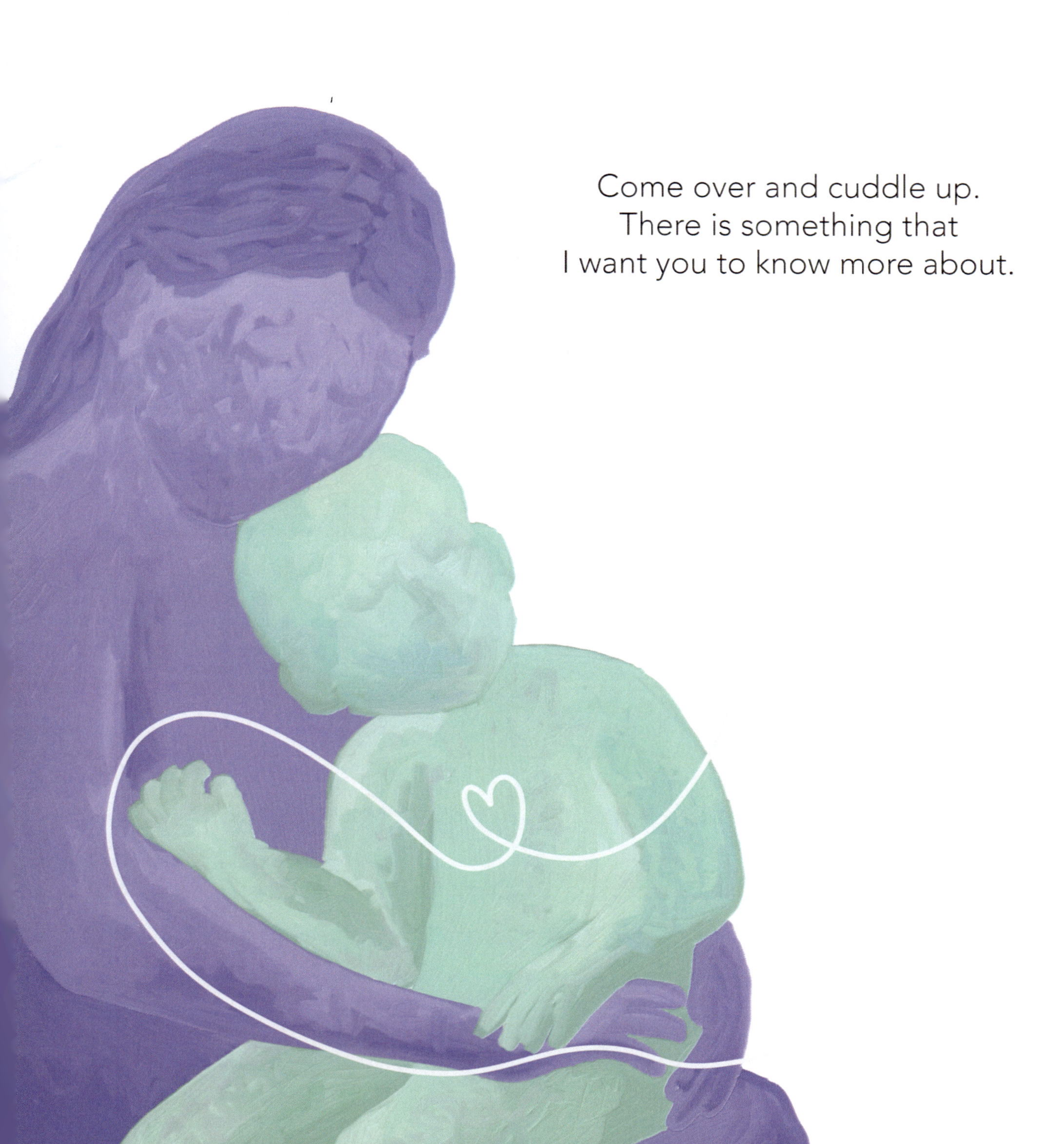

Come over and cuddle up.
There is something that
I want you to know more about.

I want you to know more about something called
maternal alloimmunization. Those are some big words, right?!
Even adults have trouble pronouncing them!

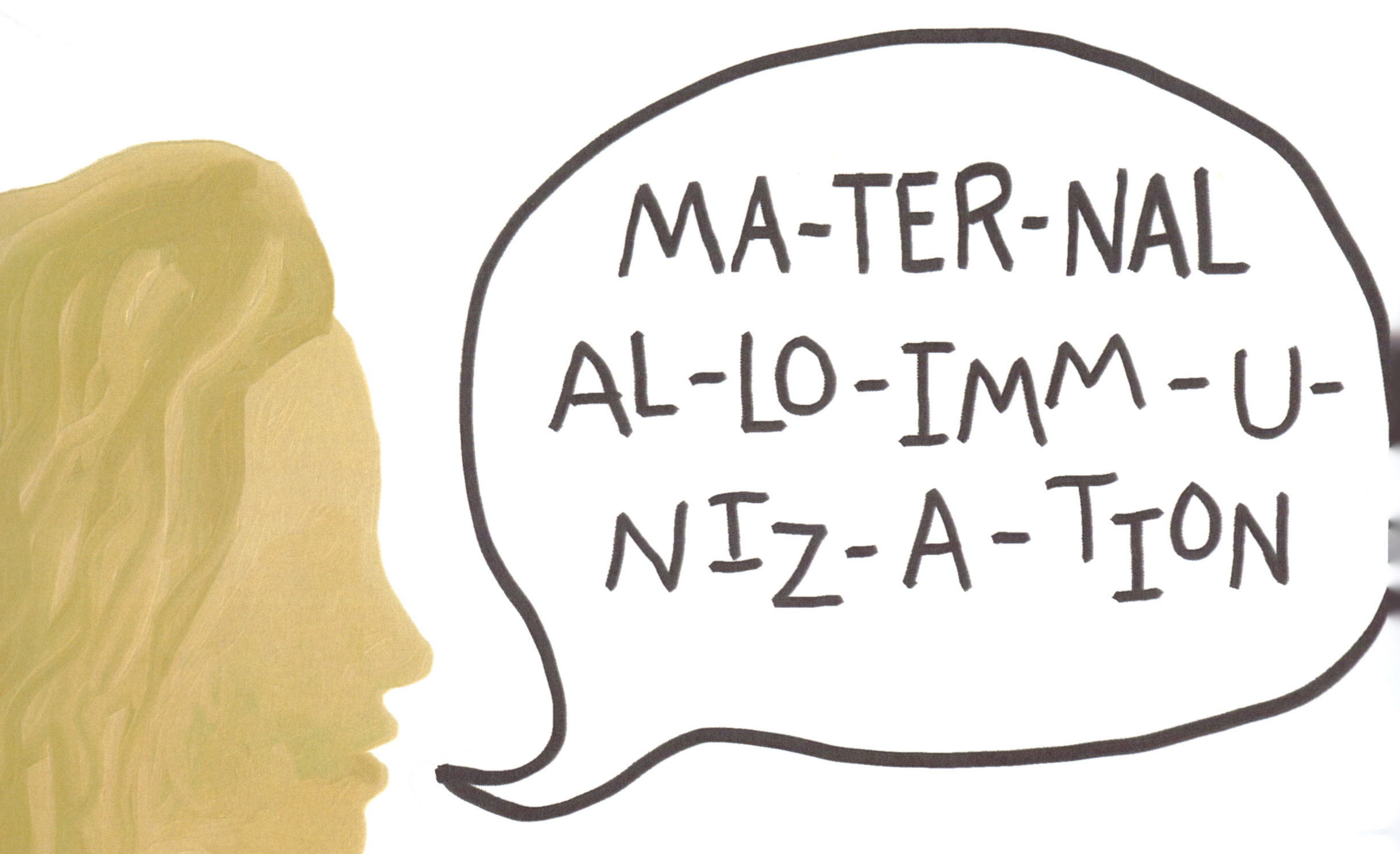

It can be hard to pronounce AND hard to explain,
but I want to try to explain because our family is a team.

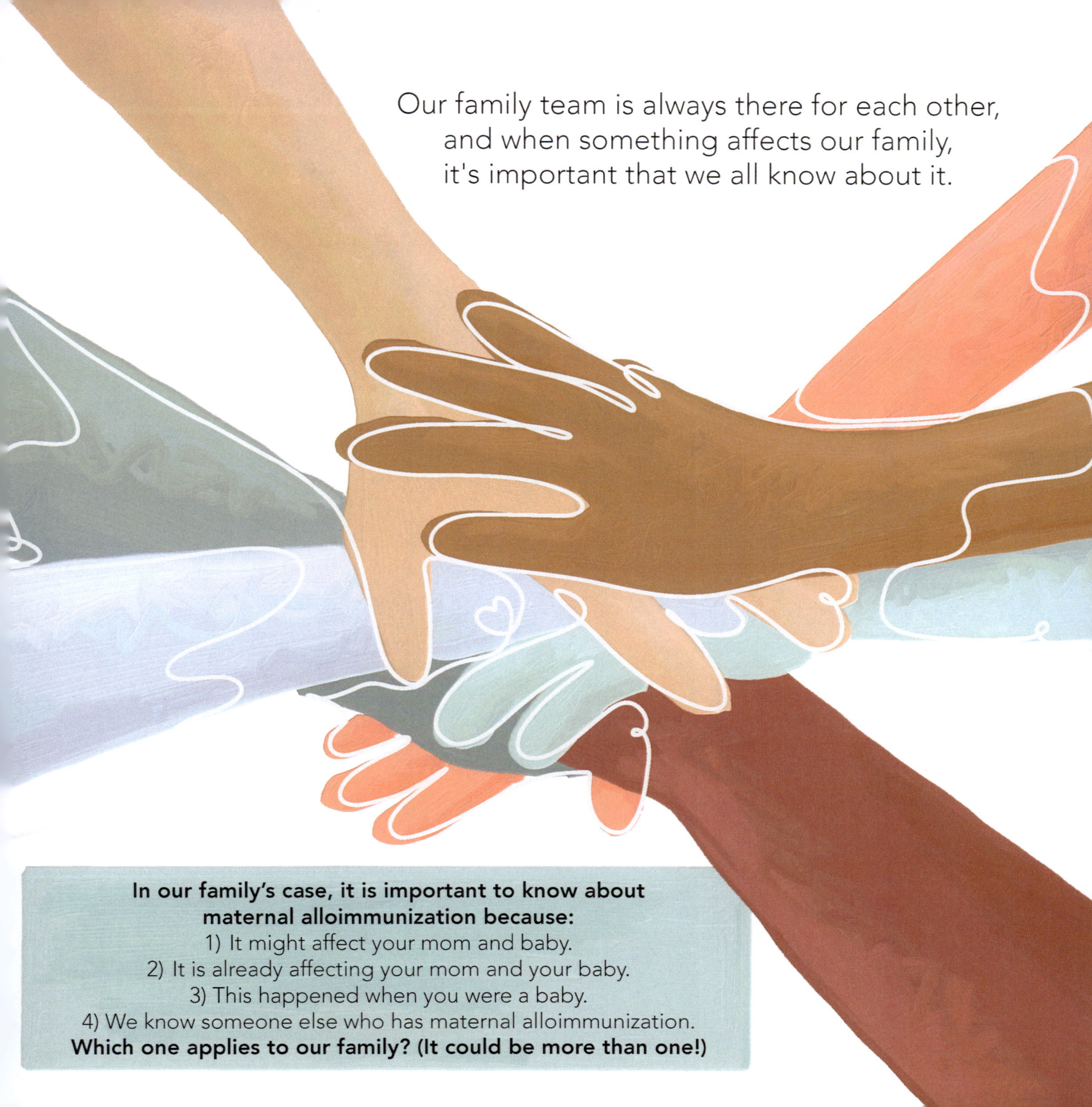

Our family team is always there for each other,
and when something affects our family,
it's important that we all know about it.

In our family's case, it is important to know about
maternal alloimmunization because:
1) It might affect your mom and baby.
2) It is already affecting your mom and your baby.
3) This happened when you were a baby.
4) We know someone else who has maternal alloimmunization.
Which one applies to our family? (It could be more than one!)

In order to understand maternal alloimmunization, it is helpful to know about immune systems. Everyone's body has an immune system, and thank goodness! Immune systems are different kinds of cells in our body that work together to keep us healthy. They fight off all sorts of things, like germs that get into our bodies and make us sick.

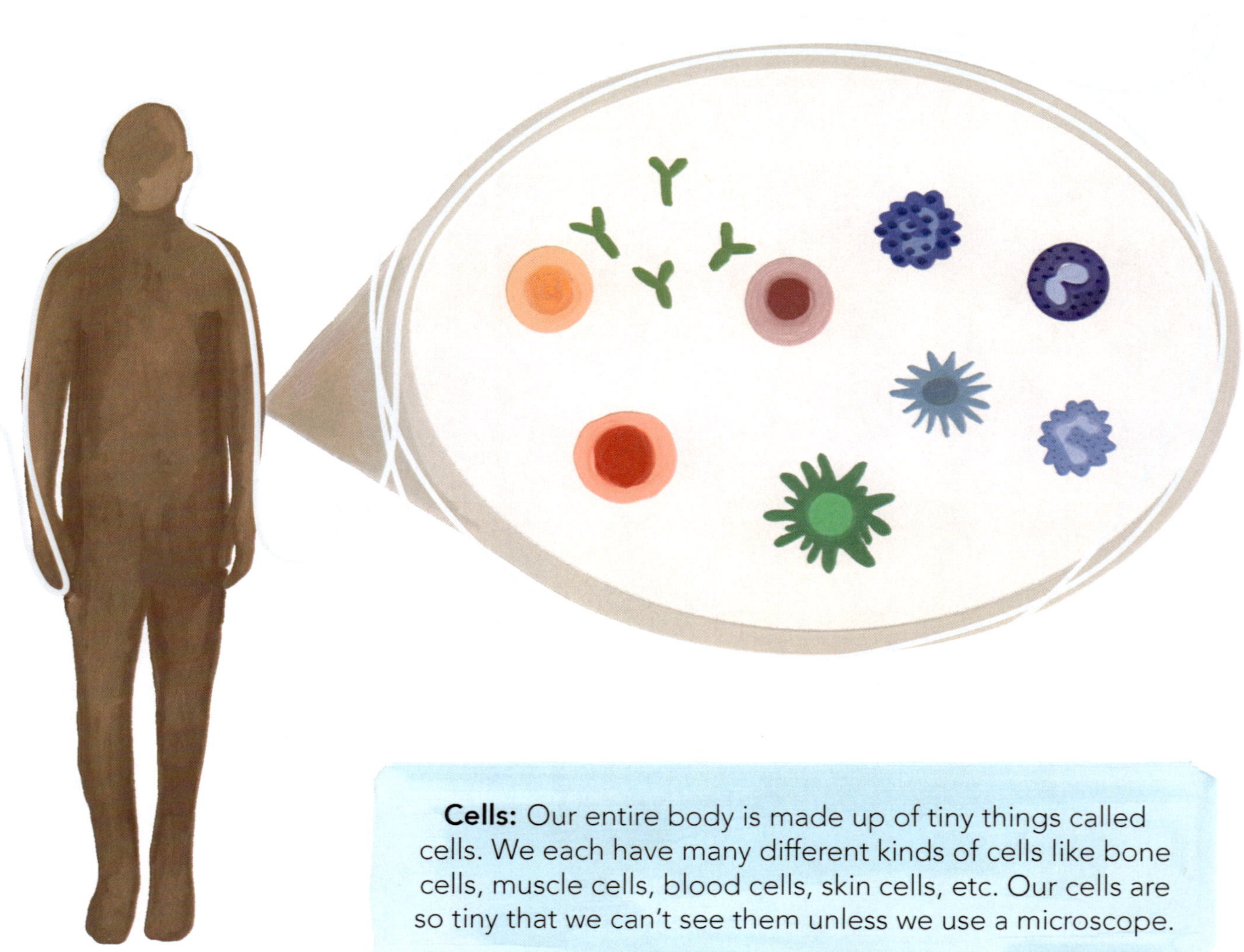

Cells: Our entire body is made up of tiny things called cells. We each have many different kinds of cells like bone cells, muscle cells, blood cells, skin cells, etc. Our cells are so tiny that we can't see them unless we use a microscope.

One amazing thing about the immune system is that it is constantly learning. Each time we are sick or a new cell type enters our body, our immune system creates an antibody that will alert the rest of the immune system if it ever sees that cell again.

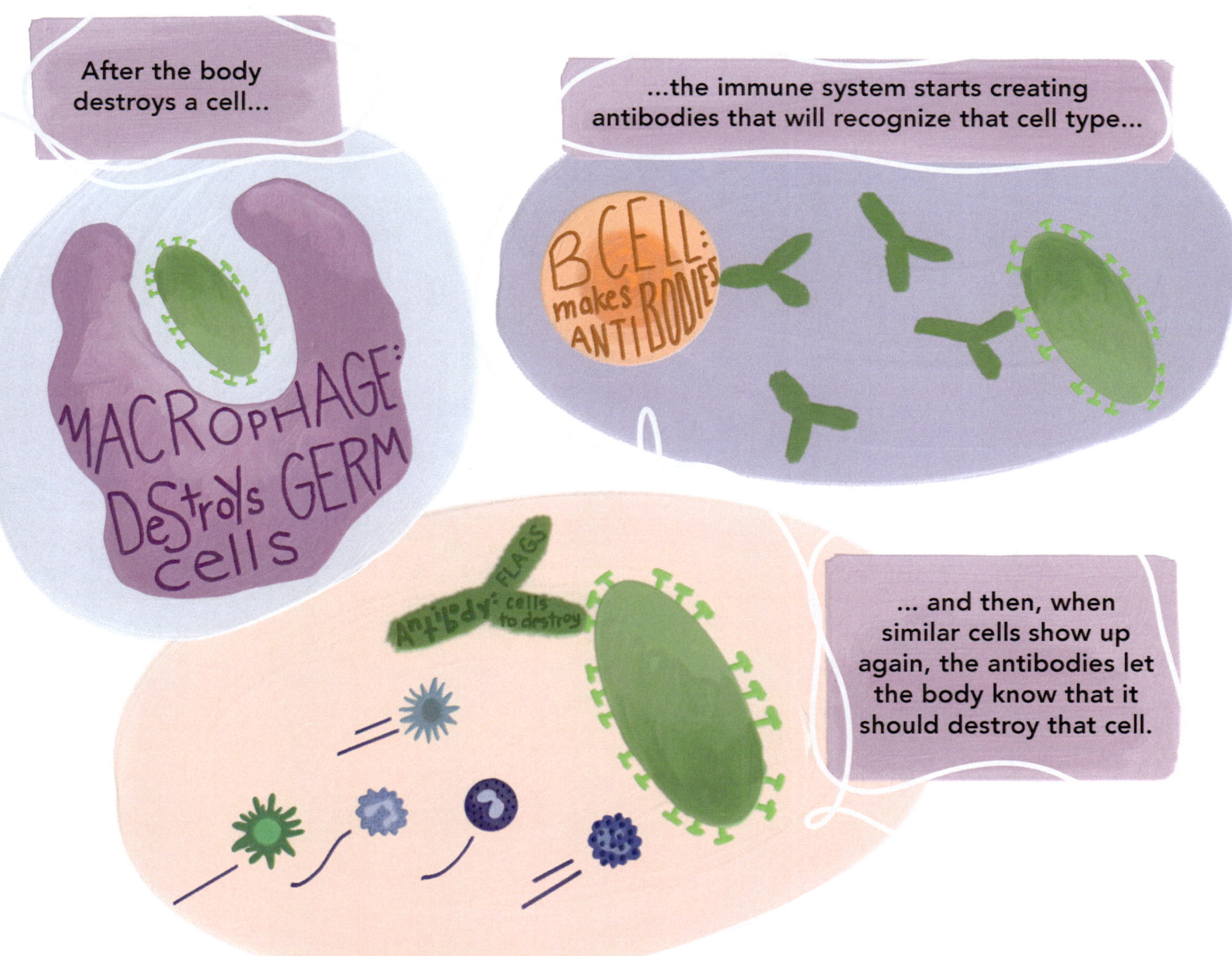

An antibody can tell that a cell is bad for the body by looking for antigens. An antigen is like a little sign that tells the antibody what kind of cell it is. If a cell has an antigen that the antibody recognizes as being bad, it attaches itself to the cell, and the rest of the immune system knows that it needs to get rid of that cell.

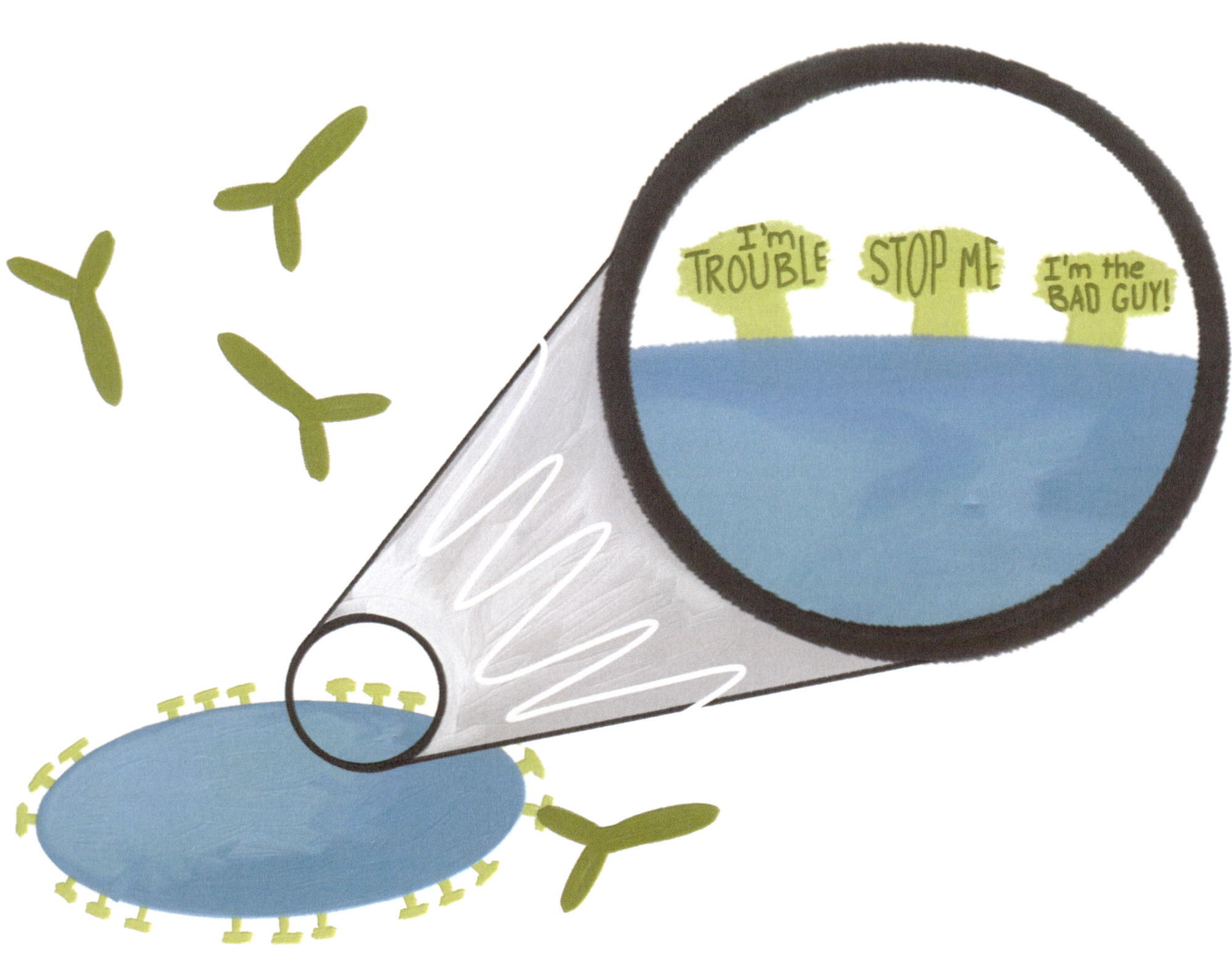

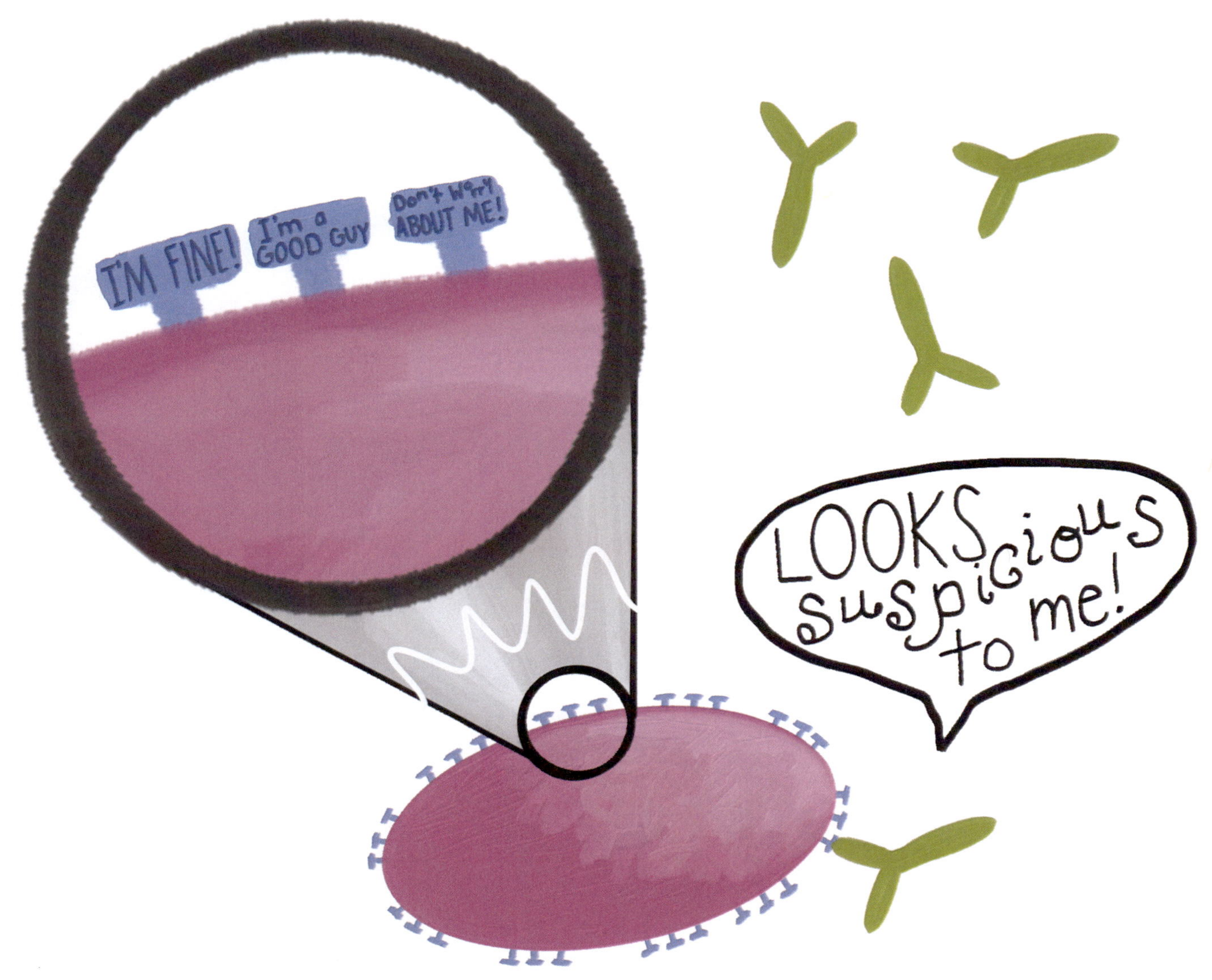

And, that's the end of the story most of the time. Except, every once in a while, the body can get rid of cells that aren't actually bad.
There can be times when the antibody decides that a new antigen is a "warning sign," when it's actually not.

There are actually quite a few different diseases that are caused by the immune system getting rid of good cells. So, doctors and scientists are getting good at finding ways to help the body when this happens.

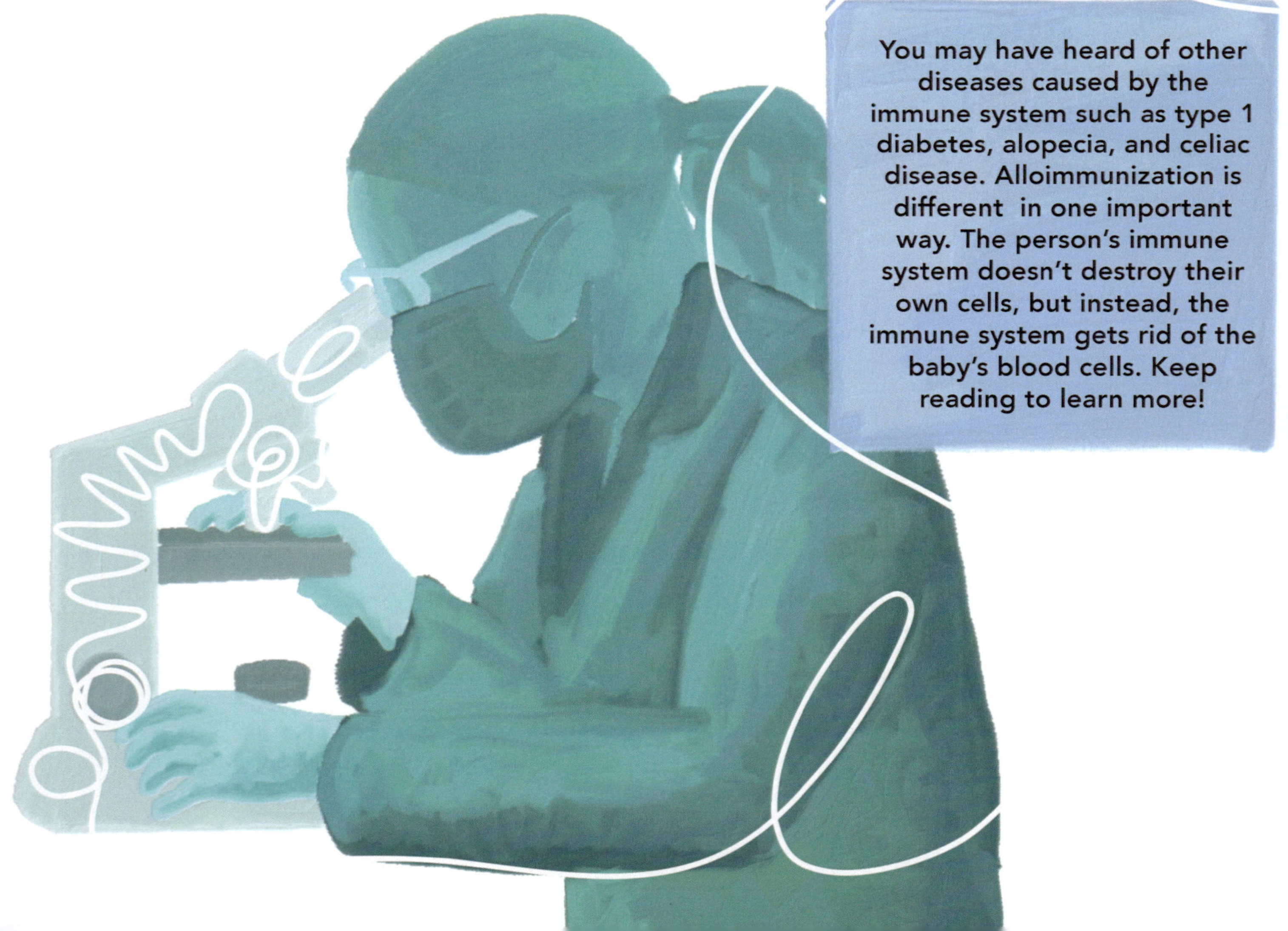

Maternal alloimmunization means a mom's immune system has made certain antibodies. These antibodies only become a problem if she becomes pregnant, and the baby's blood is different from hers. Then, these antibodies look for the baby's healthy red blood cells to break them down.

When a baby has less healthy blood cells because of the mom's antibodies, we say the baby has HDFN.
There are lots of ways we can help babies with HDFN.

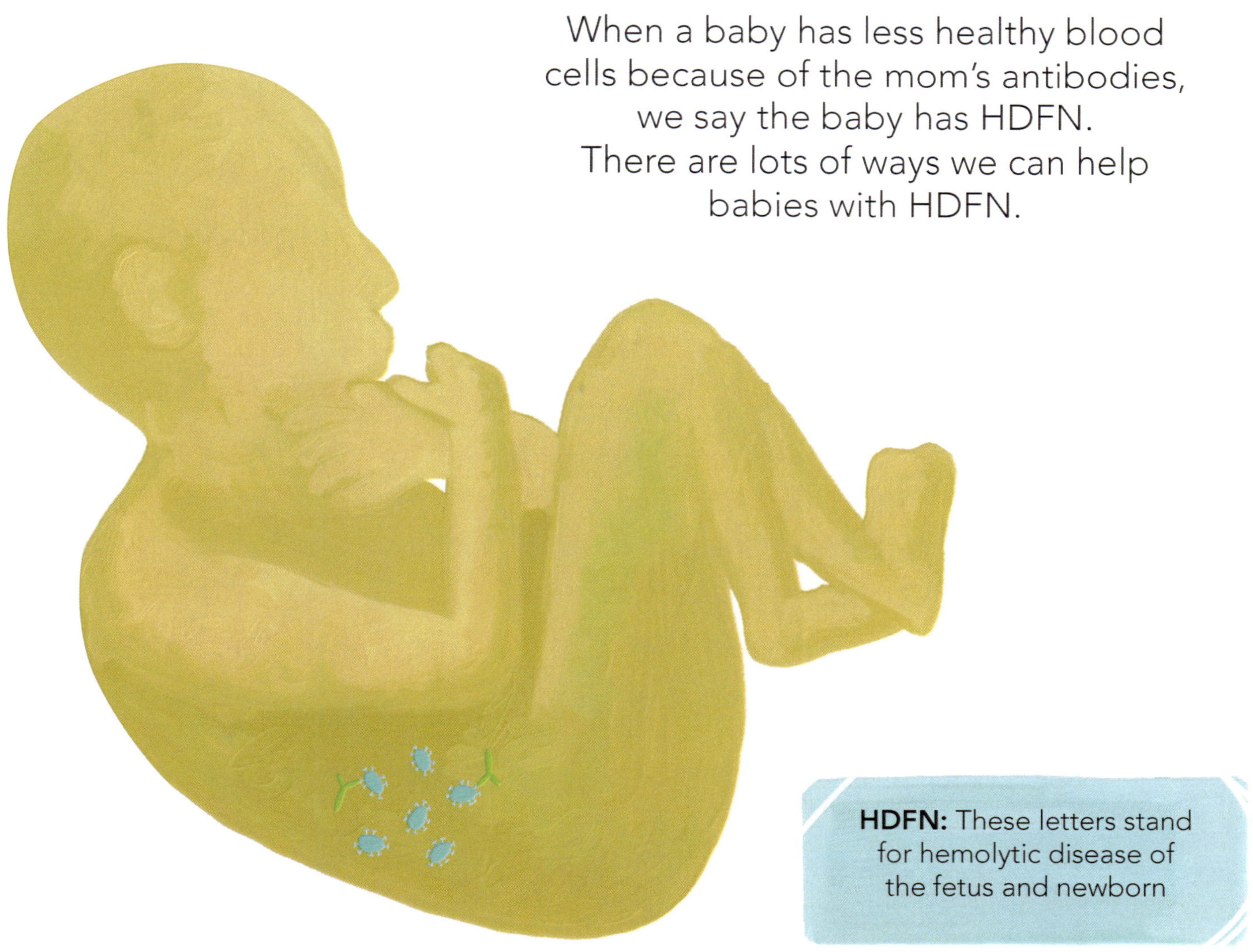

HDFN: These letters stand for hemolytic disease of the fetus and newborn

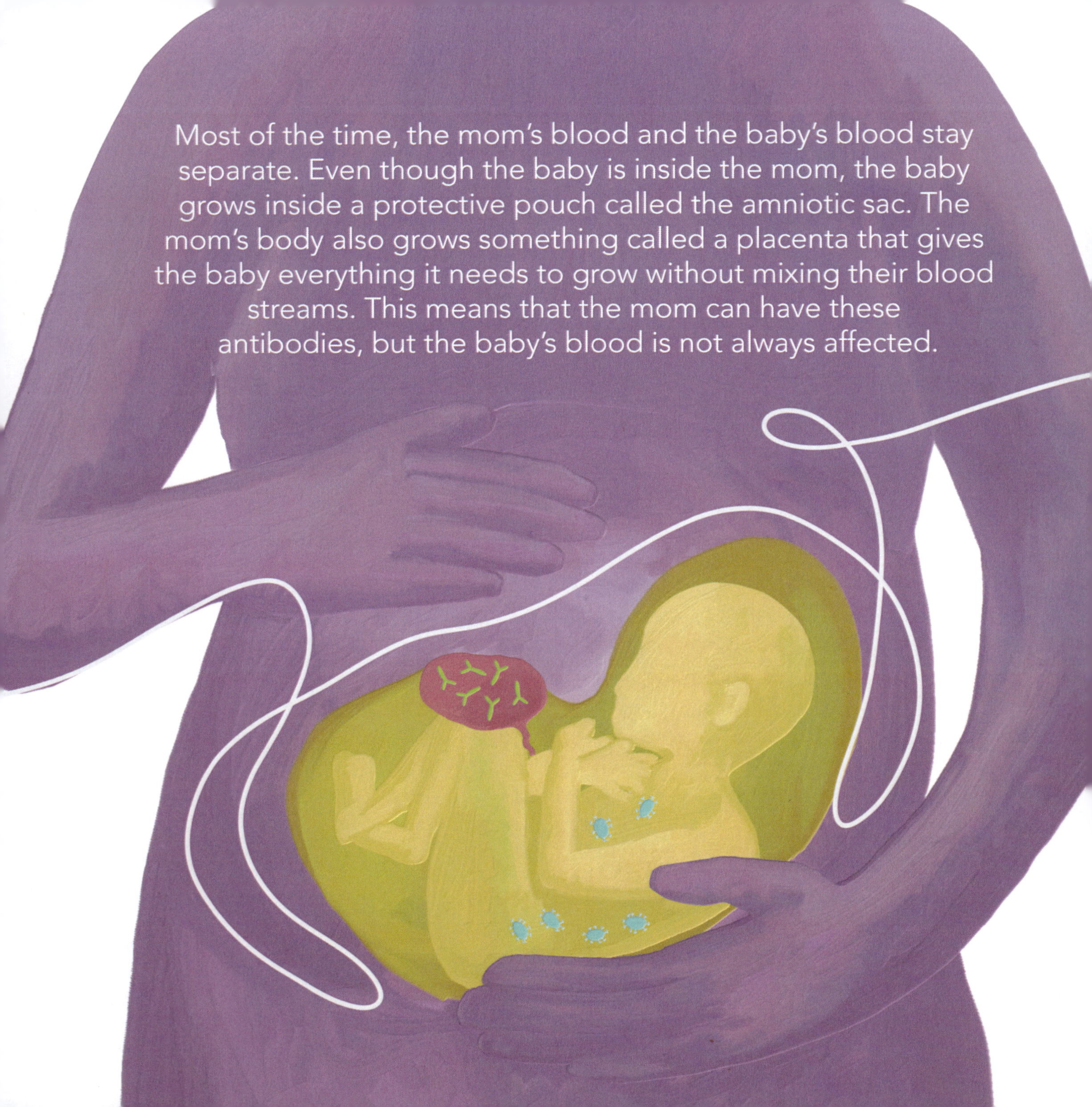

Most of the time, the mom's blood and the baby's blood stay separate. Even though the baby is inside the mom, the baby grows inside a protective pouch called the amniotic sac. The mom's body also grows something called a placenta that gives the baby everything it needs to grow without mixing their blood streams. This means that the mom can have these antibodies, but the baby's blood is not always affected.

Even though all of these things protect babies growing inside their moms, doctors still keep a close watch on moms who have the antibodies. If needed, there are so many things they can do to slow down the antibodies or to help a baby who might get HDFN.

Doctors like to be ready—just in case!

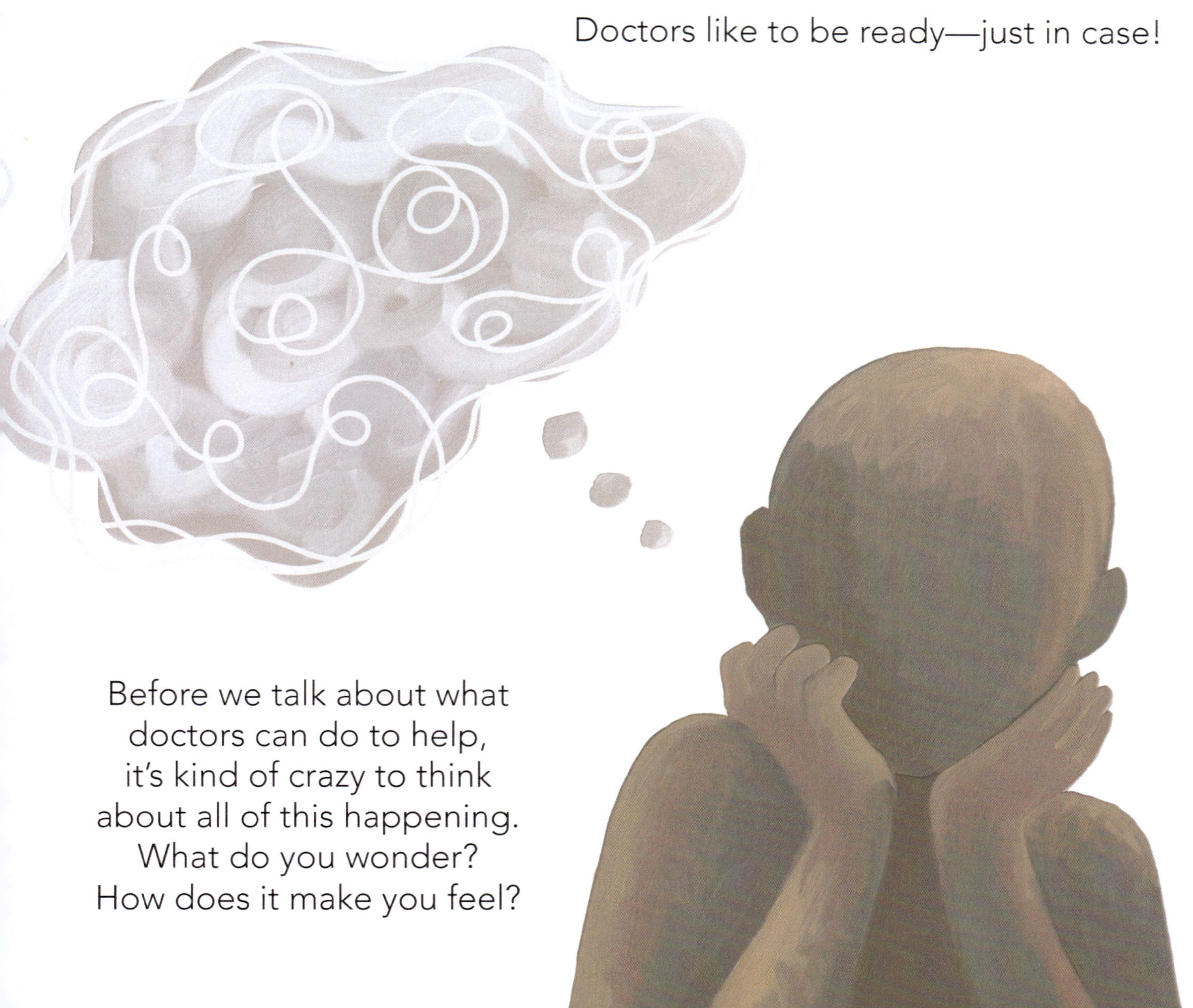

Before we talk about what doctors can do to help, it's kind of crazy to think about all of this happening. What do you wonder? How does it make you feel?

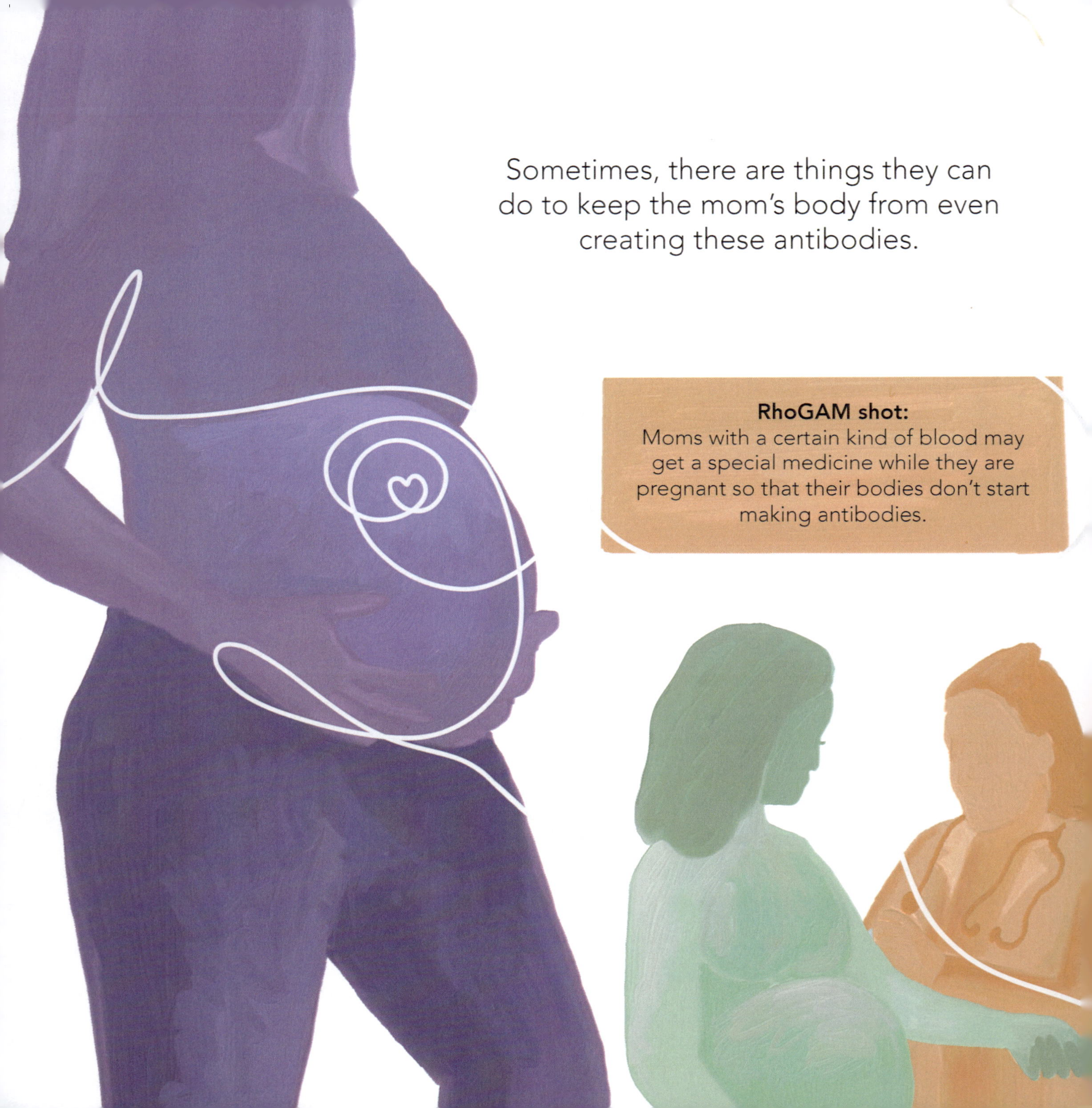

Sometimes, there are things they can do to keep the mom's body from even creating these antibodies.

When a mom has these antibodies, there are many things that can be done to help, both before and after the baby is born. Each mom and baby are different and need different things. Let's talk about all of the cool ways doctors can help!

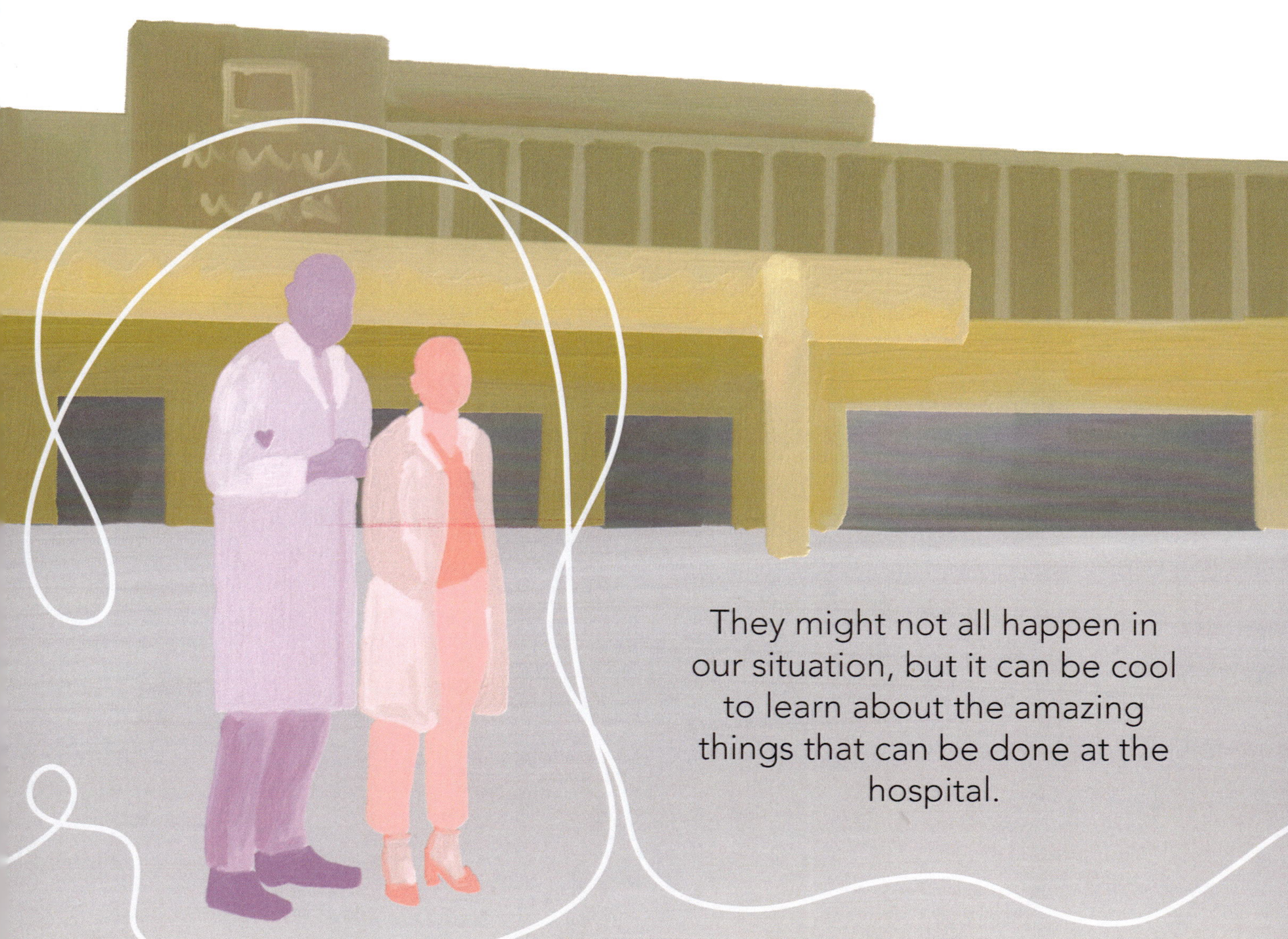

They might not all happen in our situation, but it can be cool to learn about the amazing things that can be done at the hospital.

When doctors find a lot of these antibodies in a mom's blood, there are things that hospitals can do to help. Doctors decide which kind of care will help in each situation.

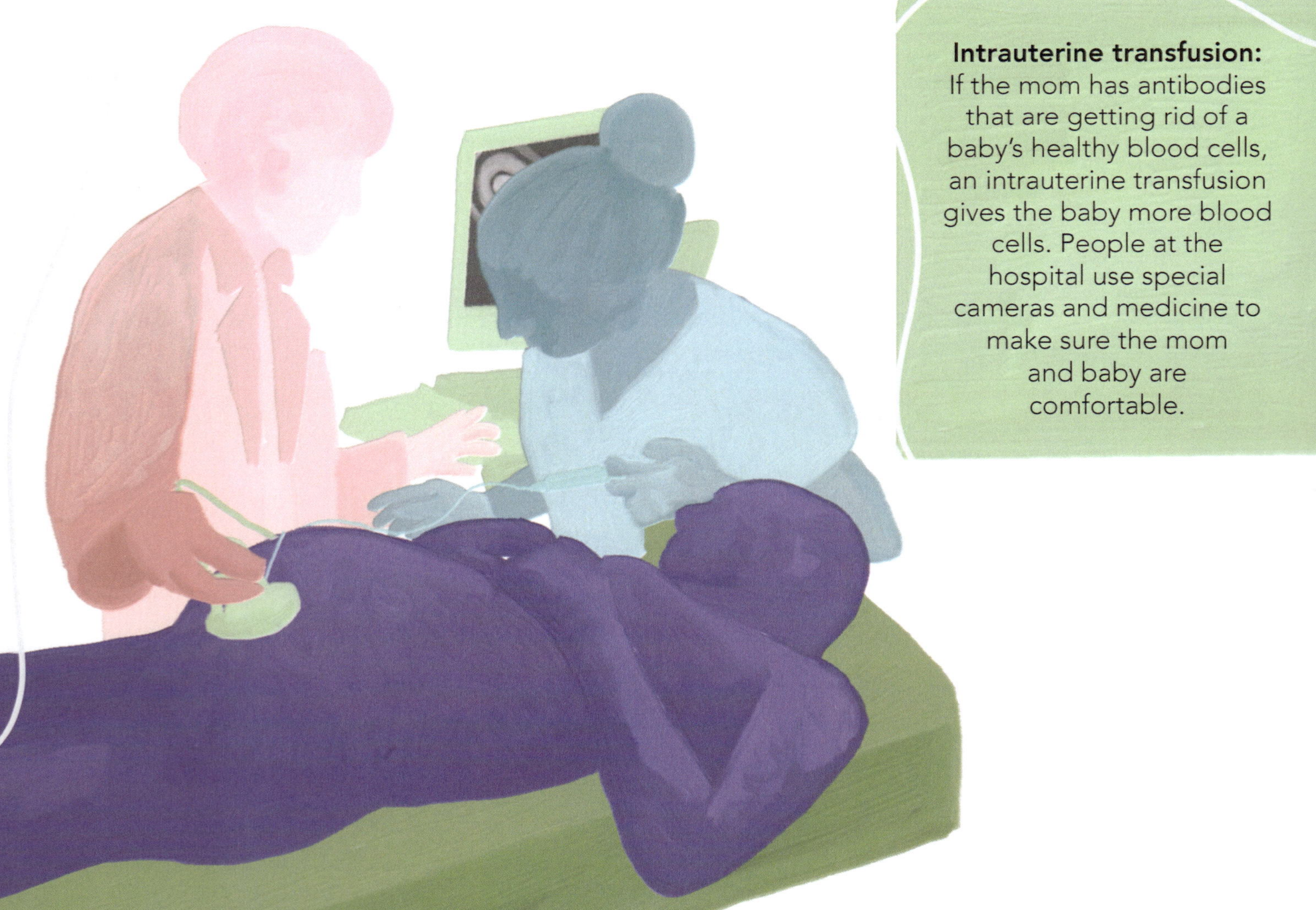

Intrauterine transfusion: If the mom has antibodies that are getting rid of a baby's healthy blood cells, an intrauterine transfusion gives the baby more blood cells. People at the hospital use special cameras and medicine to make sure the mom and baby are comfortable.

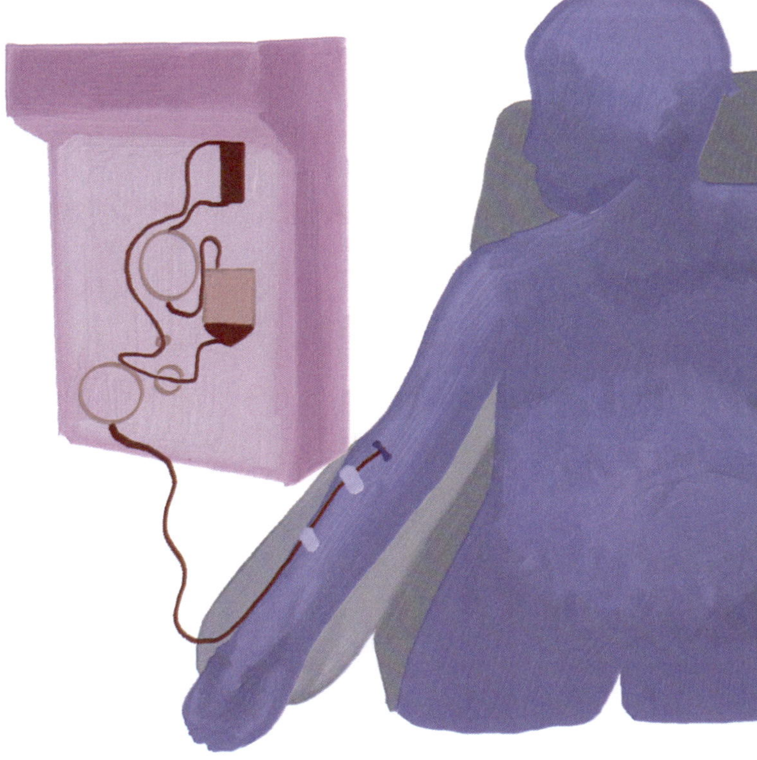

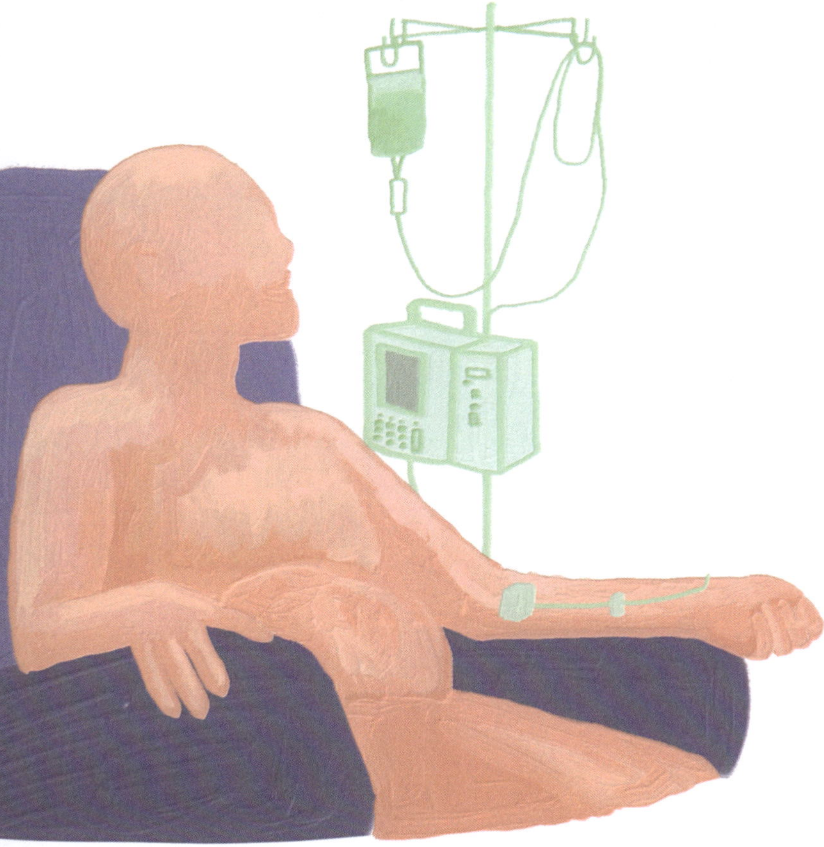

IVIG: After they find too many antibodies in a mom's blood, she gets a medicine that helps her immune system. The medicine goes into her body through an IV.

Plasmapheresis: Using an IV, the mom's blood is taken out and run through a machine that removes antibodies. Then the blood is put back into her body.

IV: A tiny straw that goes into a person's vein. Medicine can go in and blood can be taken out without having to poke someone again and again!

How do you feel about all of these things hospitals can do to help?
Do they seem a little crazy? They might make some people worry
if they have never done something like that before.

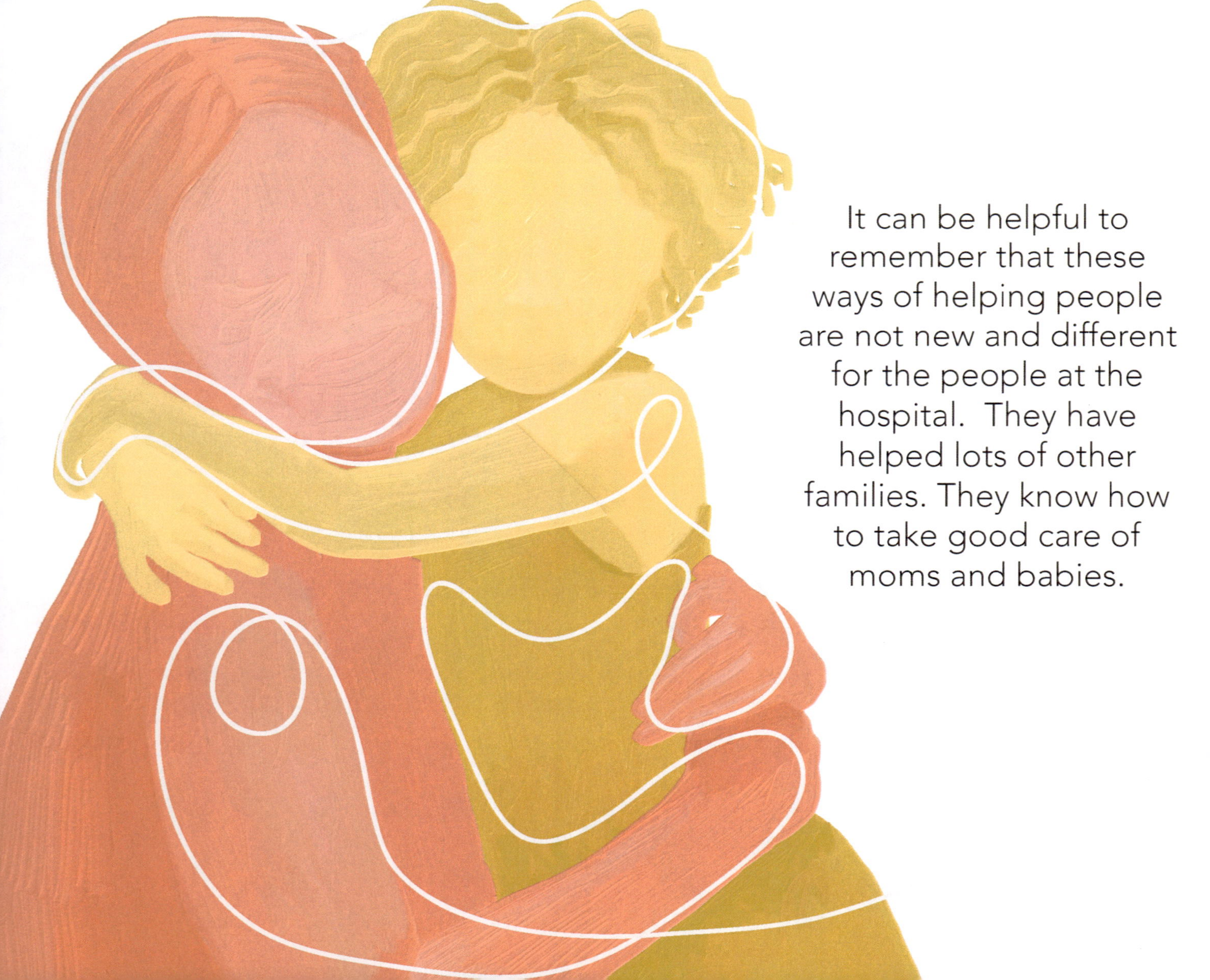

It can be helpful to
remember that these
ways of helping people
are not new and different
for the people at the
hospital. They have
helped lots of other
families. They know how
to take good care of
moms and babies.

Once the baby is born, there are more things that hospitals can do to help. The baby might not come home to live with their family right away. The baby will probably stay in a special part of the hospital where nurses and doctors carefully watch and take care of new babies.
It is called the NICU.

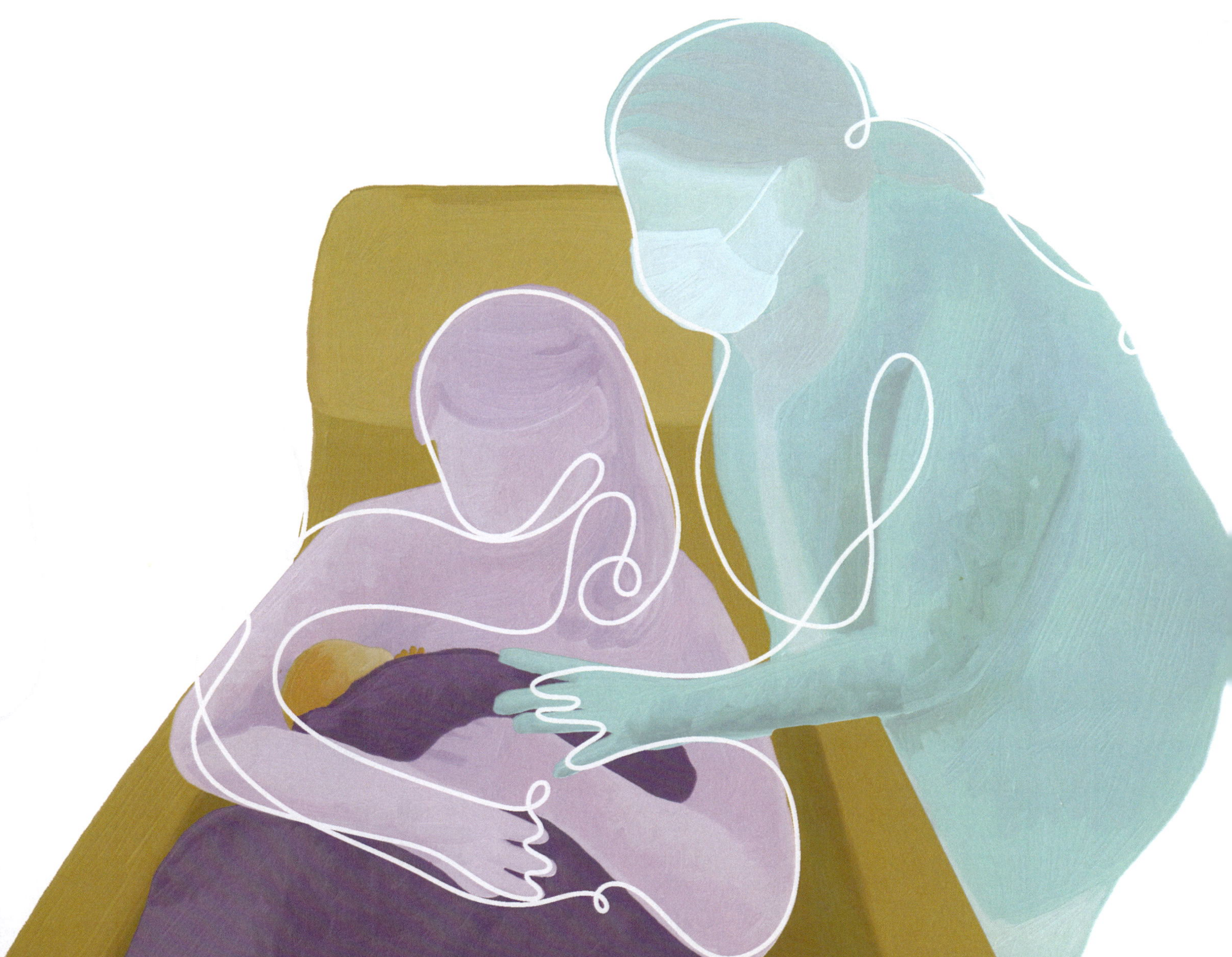

There are lots of ways doctors and nurses help babies in the NICU. Here are a few things that can help babies with HDFN:

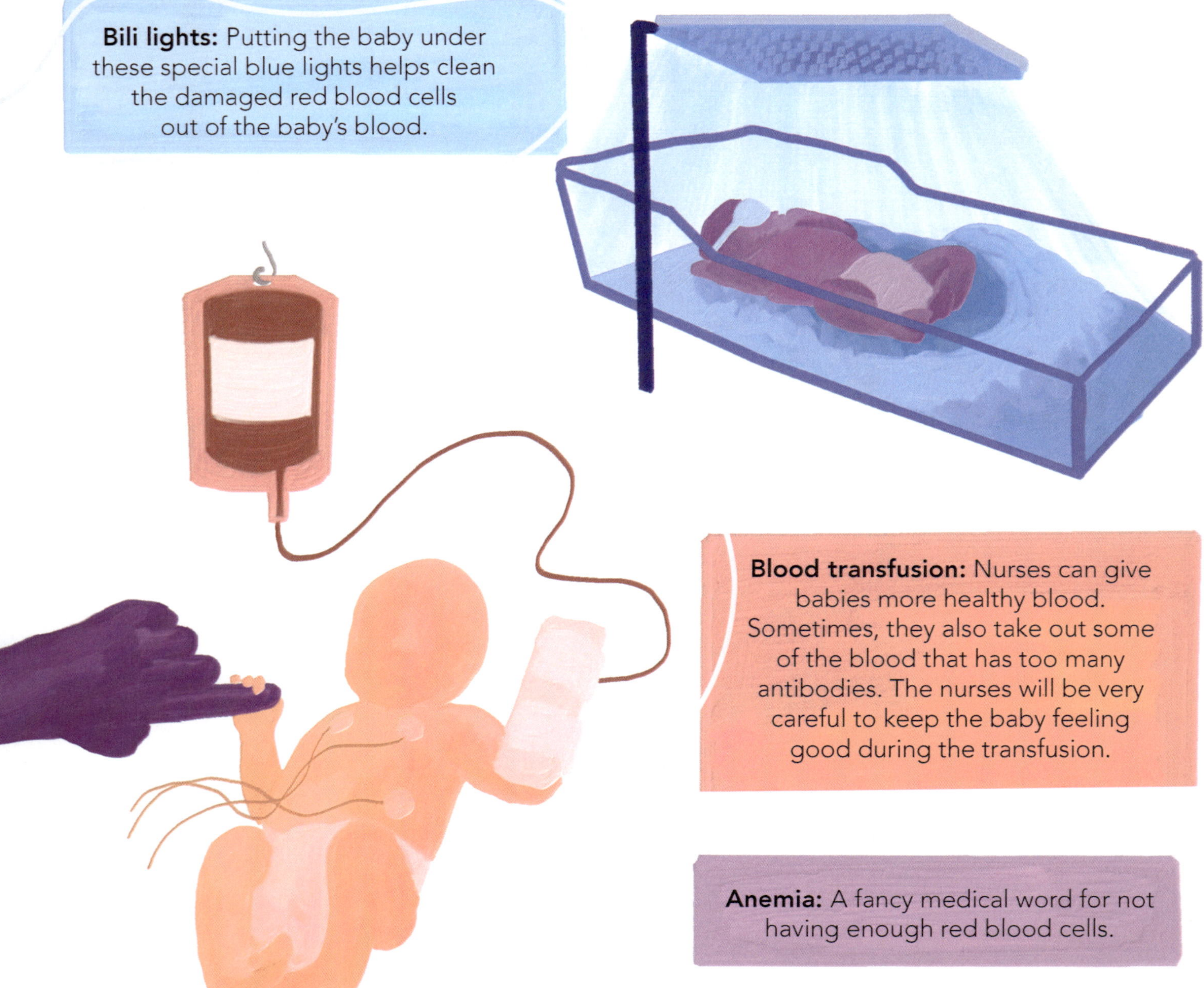

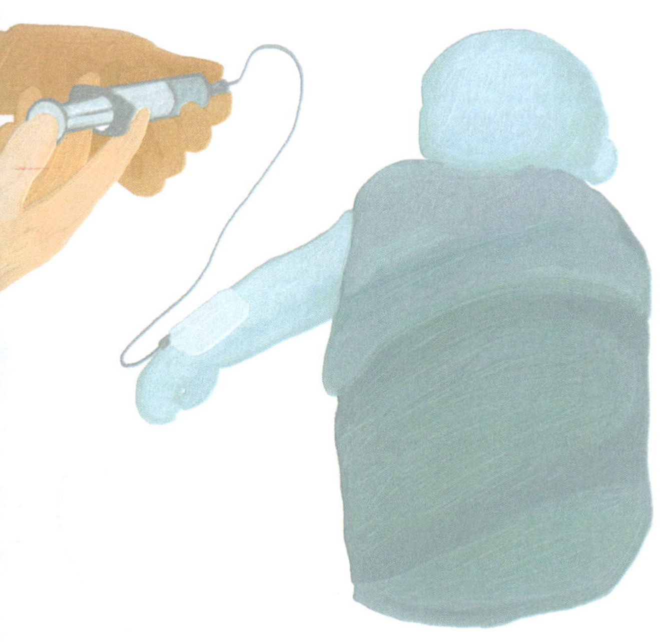

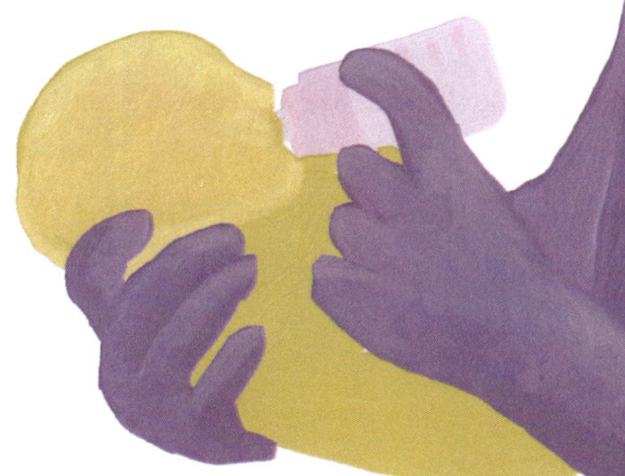

Medicine through an IV: Nurses can give the baby medicine that helps the baby's immune system and gets rid of their mom's antibodies that are still in their blood.

Feeding help: Babies who need lots of care in their first few days have trouble having enough energy to eat. In the NICU, they can give them milk through a tube in their nose or mouth until they are strong enough to be able to eat on their own.

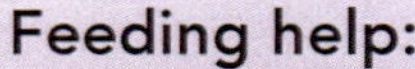

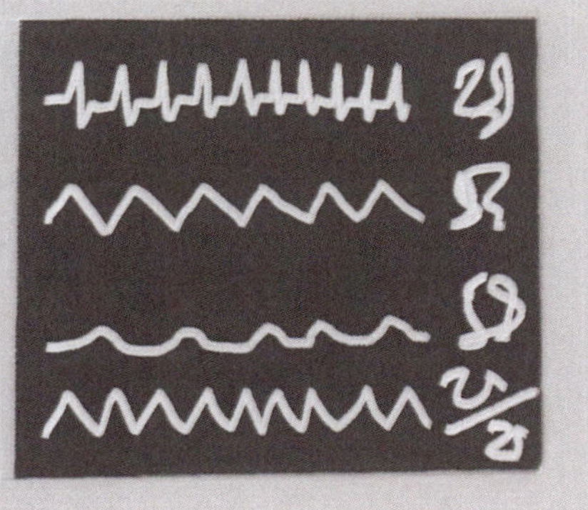

Monitors and vitals: When babies are in the NICU, they can't use words to tell people when something isn't right. Instead, each baby wears stickers that measure their heartbeat and their breathing. The stickers send the measurements to a computer that can show nurses, doctors, and parents how the baby's body is doing. Sometimes, the computer might beep. This means that the computer has noticed a change and a parent or a nurse might need to check it out.

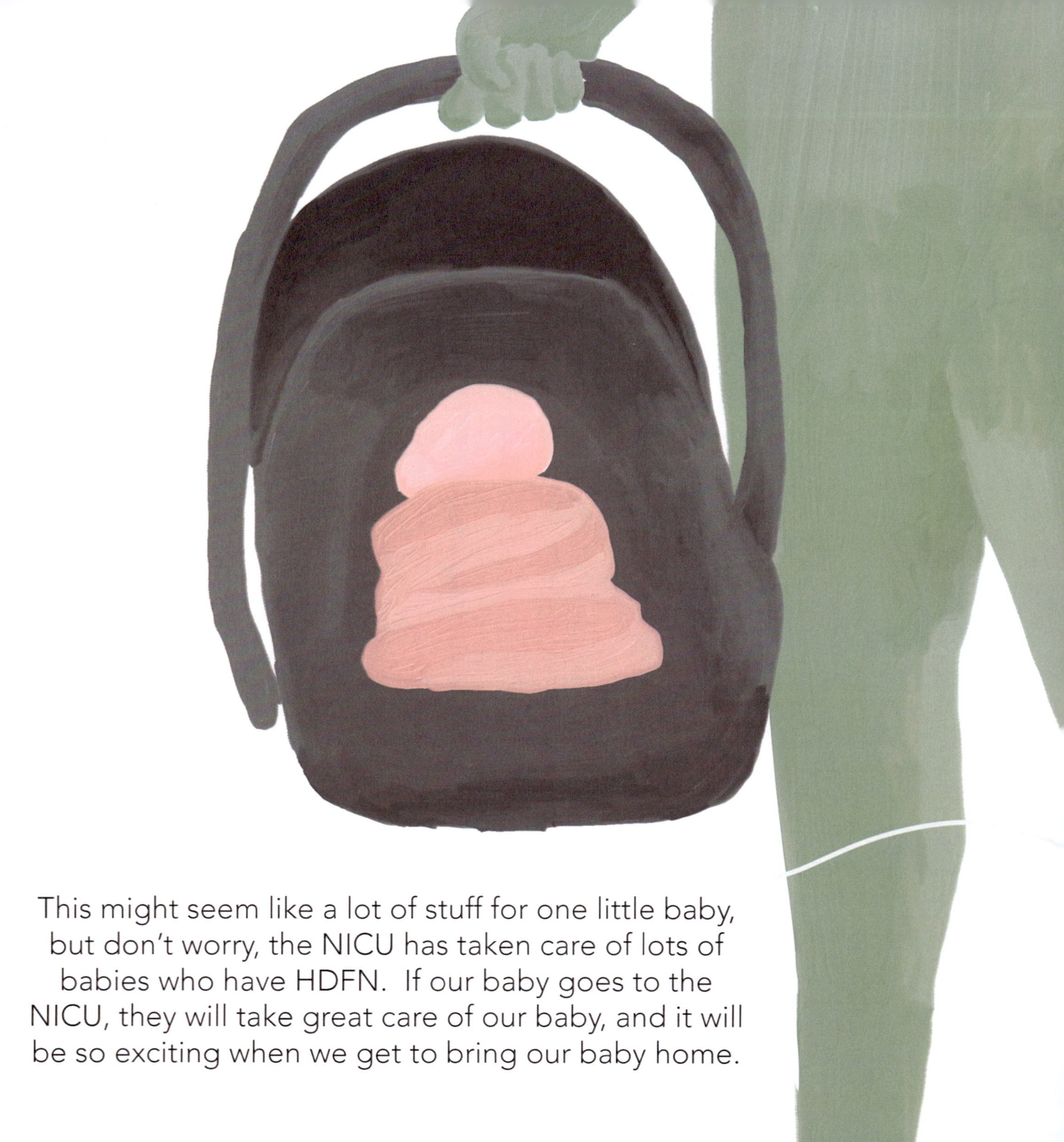

This might seem like a lot of stuff for one little baby, but don't worry, the NICU has taken care of lots of babies who have HDFN. If our baby goes to the NICU, they will take great care of our baby, and it will be so exciting when we get to bring our baby home.

The people in the NICU have to be very careful. They wash their hands a lot and wear special clothes so that they don't bring germs to the new baby. They have to talk quietly and be very gentle. New babies who have HDFN need lots of rest so that their body can work on growing red blood cells and learning to drink milk.

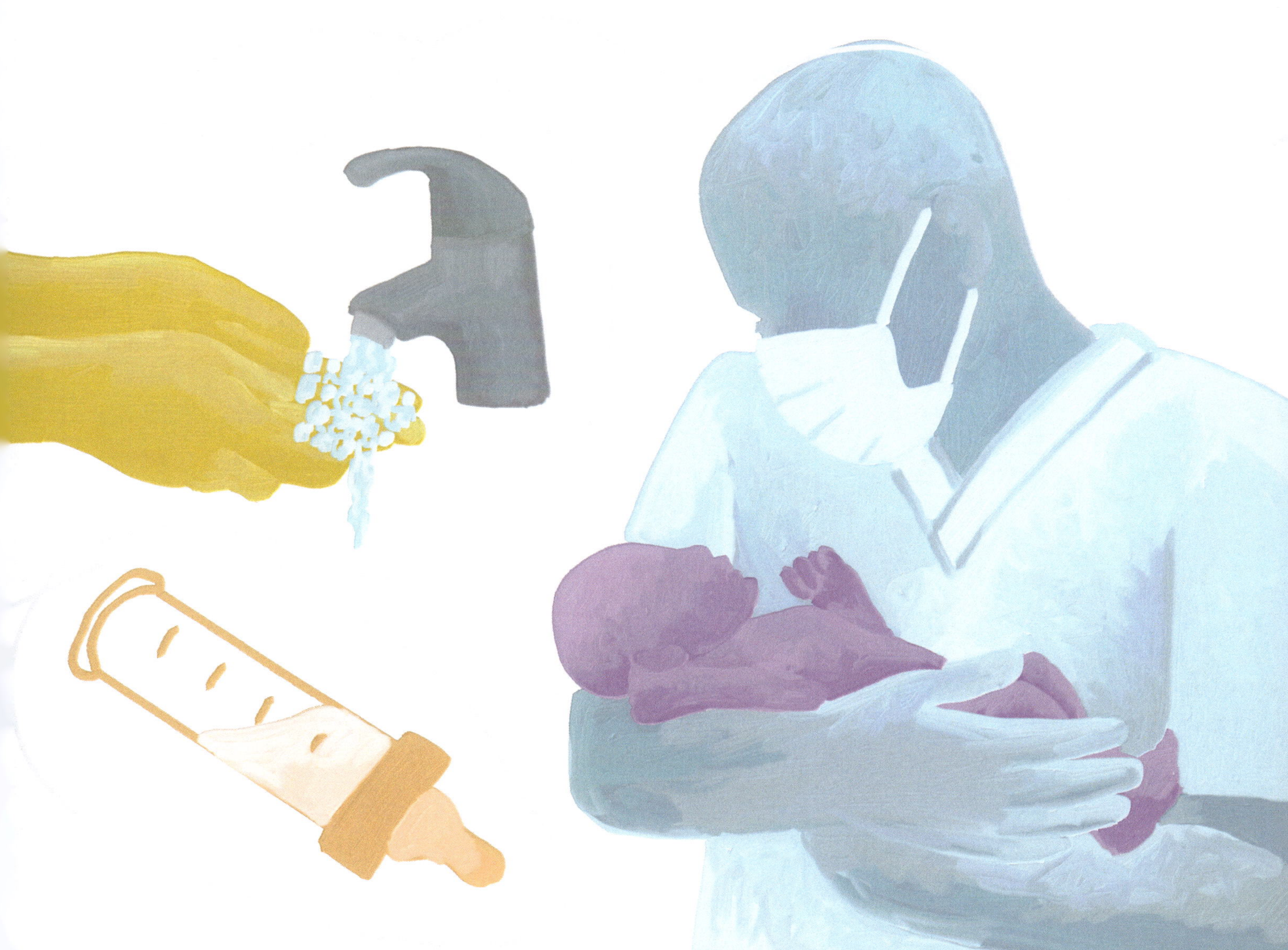

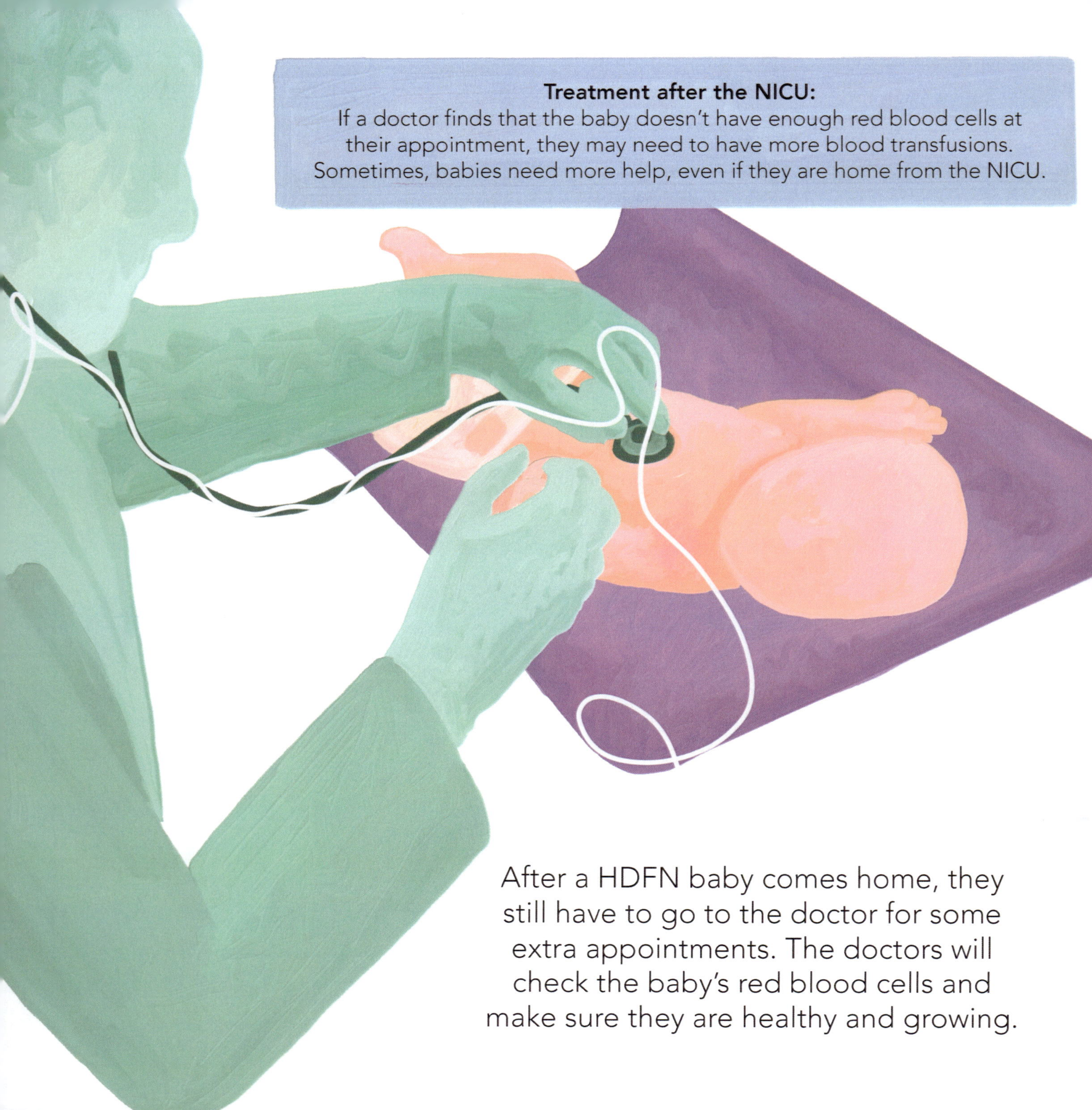

After a HDFN baby comes home, they still have to go to the doctor for some extra appointments. The doctors will check the baby's red blood cells and make sure they are healthy and growing.

Now, here is another crazy part. Even though
HDFN babies need all this extra care,
HDFN is over pretty quickly. Most babies
don't need any more extra care by the time
they are four months old.

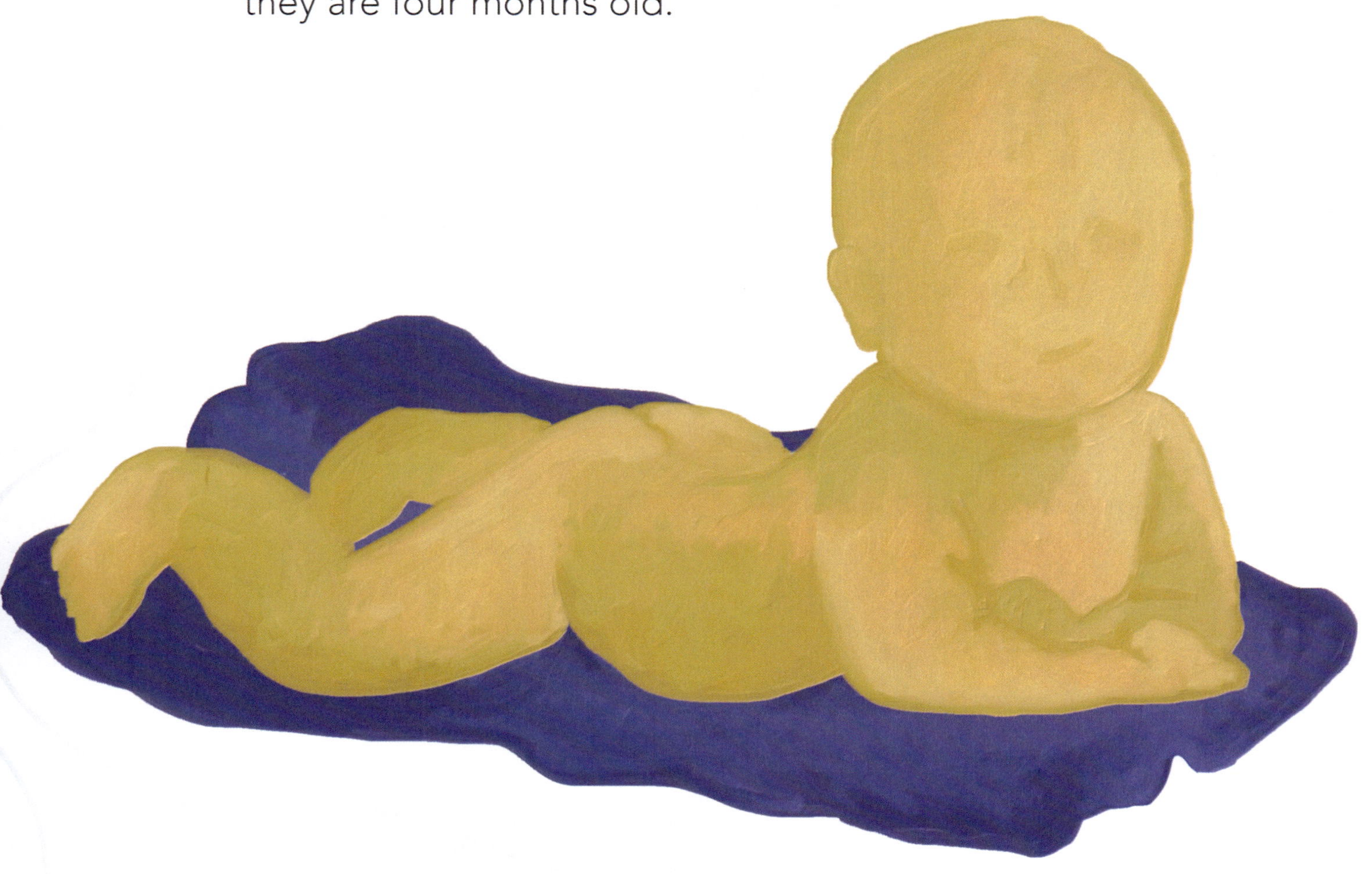

As the baby grows up, most people will never
even know that this happened.

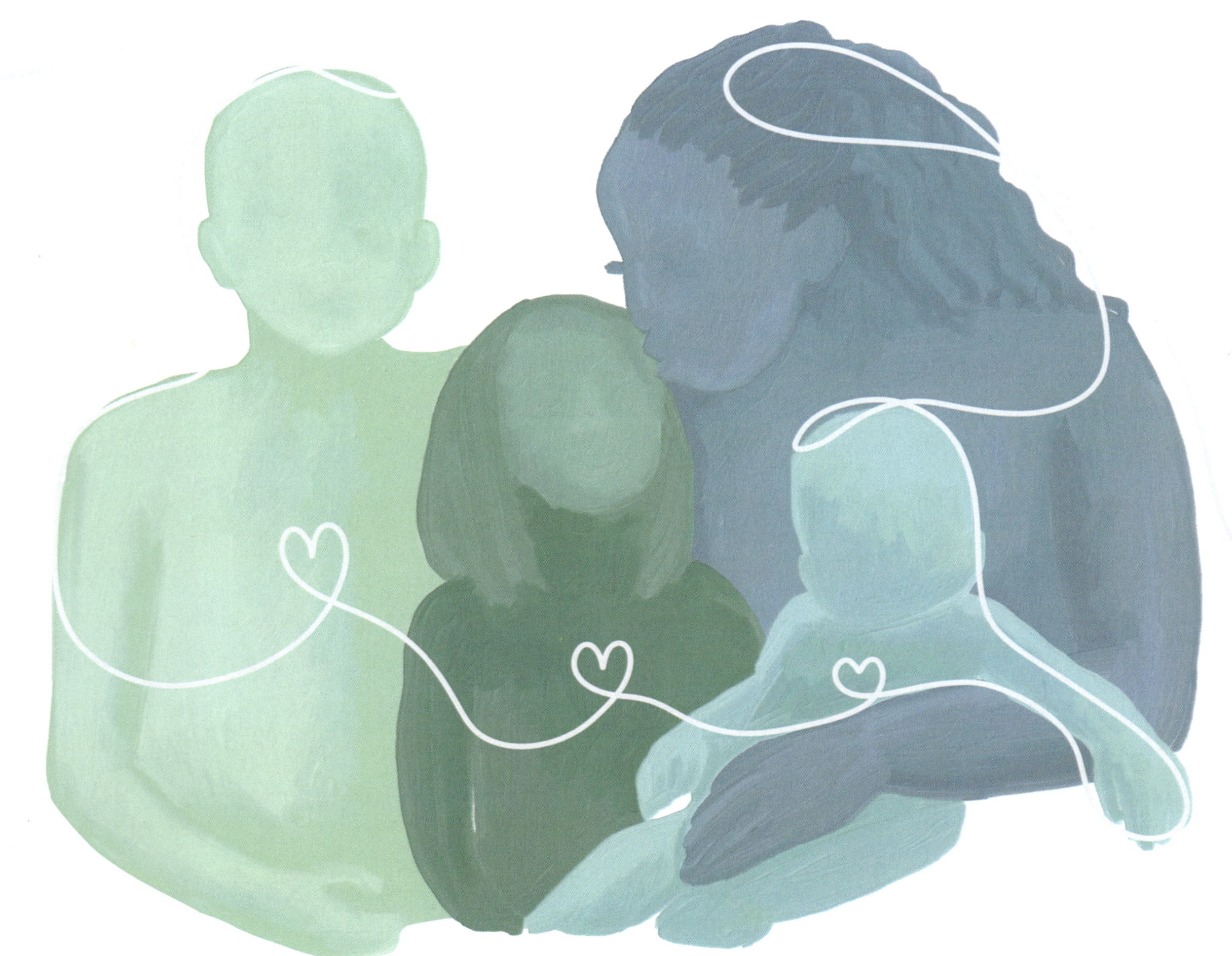

In some families, this only happens with one pregnancy.
In other families, a mom might have this happen over and
over. She might have more than one pregnancy
affected by maternal alloimmunization.

As each baby grows, they won't remember all of this. Some day, they may need to read this book to learn about all of the special care they got when they were tiny. It will be just one tiny thing that makes them unique.

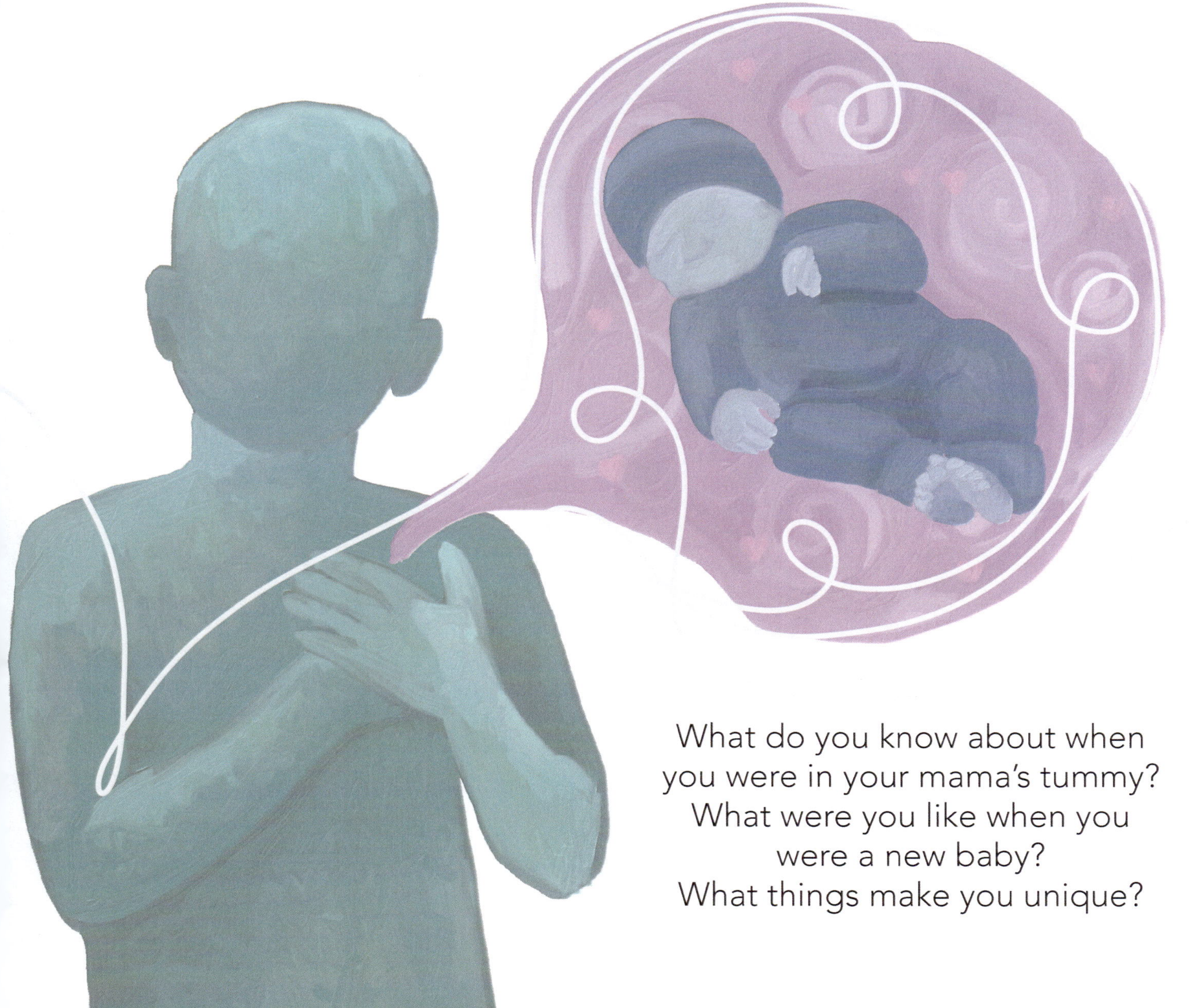

What do you know about when
you were in your mama's tummy?
What were you like when you
were a new baby?
What things make you unique?

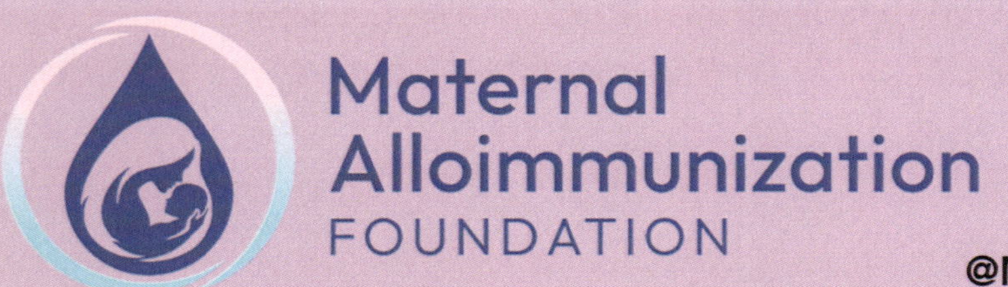

www.alloimmunization.org
www.HDFN.org

Instagram: @alloimmunization
Facebook:
@MaternalAlloimmunizationFoundation

The Maternal Alloimmunization Foundation is a patient-led nonprofit that stands beside families facing maternal alloimmunization and the newborn condition it can cause, called hemolytic disease of the fetus and newborn (HDFN). MAF raises awareness, educates patients and providers, and works to improve care for both moms and babies.
We hope this book helps do all of these things too.

We'd love to support you in any way possible. Connect with our community on socials, and learn more about alloimmunization, HDFN, and our organization on our website (listed above).

Words Worth Repeating

www.wordsworthrepeating.com

Facebook: @WordsWorthRepeatingBooks
Instagram: @words.worth.repeating
YouTube: Words Worth Repeating

Words Worth Repeating is an organization that empowers families to have hard and important conversations by creating books that give families the gentle, yet honest words.

Words Worth Repeating children's books are written by a child life specialist and include colorful inclusive illustrations. Words Worth Repeating partners with non-profits who are passionate and excited about giving families thoughtful resources. In addition, Words Worth Repeating creates customizable books and templates for families who want to create a book about their own unique situation, diagnosis, or loved one.

Learn more about all of these resources on the website, and connect with Laura as she promotes supporting families through children's books on her socials (listed above).

9 798992 101287